# NATURAL ❧REMEDIES❧

# Colds<sup>for</sup> & Flu

**HOW TO BOOST YOUR IMMUNE SYSTEM, PROTECT YOURSELF
NATURALLY AND PREVENT COLDS AND INFLUENZA WITH
HERBAL REMEDIES AND EASY LIFESTYLE CHANGES**

Copyright © 2014 Kasia Roberts, RN
All right reserved.

# Disclaimer

*The information in this book is not to be used as medical advice and is not meant to treat or diagnose medical problems. The information presented should be used in combination with guidance from your physician.*

*All rights reserved. No part of this publication or the information in it may be quoted from or reproduced in any form by means such as printing, scanning, photocopying or otherwise without prior written permission of the copyright holder.*

*Disclaimer and Terms of Use: Effort has been made to ensure that the information in this book is accurate and complete, however, the author and the publisher do not warrant the accuracy of the information, text and graphics contained within the book due to the rapidly changing nature of science, research, known and unknown facts and internet. The Author and the publisher do not hold any responsibility for errors, omissions or contrary interpretation of the subject matter herein. This book is presented solely for motivational and informational purposes only.*

## Introduction

It's three a.m. in the morning and you can't fall asleep. You have difficulty breathing. You feel aches and pains in your body, you're chilled to the bone and even your cat is beginning to dislike you as you sneeze again and again reaching for more tissues. Are you likely to die? Most likely not, although the villain, the common cold or flu, can certainly make you feel as if you're on your death bed.

We've all been sick with a cold or flu at one time or another but is it necessary to keep getting sick? How can we protect ourselves naturally in order to fight off pathogens and viruses we may come in contact with? How many events or workdays have you missed as a result of the common cold or flu? If you're anything like the typical person, you've missed quite a few. Cold and flu symptoms: coughs, sniffles, headaches, body aches, and fever greatly reduce our productivity and leave us feeling exhausted and tired. There is good news however, you can rise above them utilizing tried and true herbal techniques, natural remedies and simple lifestyle changes that will enable you to supercharge your immune system and protect you from the cold and flu virus—techniques that look to the bountiful energy of the earth for richness and vibrant health.

As we all know, the common cold and flu are different from each other; the cold, on its own, doesn't sound too malignant. However, the flu can rise to another level—knocking people out for ten days or more. You can learn to protect yourself naturally through altering your lifestyle habits, for example, learning not to touch stair railings and getting in the habit of washing your hands and sanitizing with alcohol as you go through your day-to-day life. More importantly, it's better to begin addressing your health from the inside. Learn about the incredibly beneficial vitamin D: the vitamin your body creates every time you stand in the sunshine. If you get enough vitamin D in your system, you automatically boost your immune system and halt future flu and cold symptoms. What's more? Vitamin D has been proven to be more efficient in reducing your affinity for disease than the common flu vaccine.

The controversial topic of the flu vaccine is also addressed in this book. The hidden agenda of doctors and pharmaceutical companies, spouting their belief the in the flu vaccine and encouraging the public to get the flu shot, can become a little alarming. Learn the facts for yourself and discover if you actually want to seek the flu vaccine for yourself and your children. You will be surprised at what hidden chemicals the flu vaccine actually contains.

Learn to live a better, more vibrant, healthy day-to-day life. Learn about the five top-tier herbal remedies to boost your immune system and fight back against disease; furthermore, learn 8 herbal and essential oil-based remedies to calm your symptoms when you do fall ill.

Remember the benefits of living a calm, less stressed, more active, and happier life. You can reduce your flu and cold risks; you can fuel yourself with relief; and you can turn to natural, herbal remedies whenever you're feeling a little under-the-weather for rapid relief. Learn to become self-sustaining, and never miss another life event again due to the cold or flu.

# Table of Contents

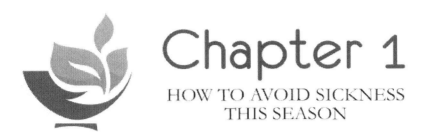

# Chapter 1
## HOW TO AVOID SICKNESS THIS SEASON

It's winter. As the weather drops to drastic low temperatures, you're likely concerned with holiday plans, decorating, shopping—everything delightful and joyous about this otherwise chilly and dreadful time of year. Unfortunately, as you fly through the obstacles of the holiday season and wind your way through crowded mall hallways, you're putting yourself at greater and greater risk of developing colds and flu. This is the most contagious time of year: the time of year when you're quite likely to pick an illness and fall flat on your bed for a week or so. As such, it's essential that you educate yourself about this cold and flu season, understand the symptoms, and learn how to heal yourself naturally.

## Differences between Cold and Flu

This "most wonderful time of the year" of cold and flu brings scratchy throats, stuffed noses, and constant headaches. However, cold and flu symptoms can be quite similar, forcing you into a state of confusion. How do you know which you have? Because flu is much more serious than the cold, it's important to understand the differences.

## What is the Common Cold?

The cold is referred to as the "common" cold because—well—nearly everyone suffers from it, at one time or another. It is the single most "common" reason people head to their doctor's office during the year; it's the most common reason people miss work and school, as well. Symptoms of the common cold usually last around fourteen days; these symptoms are generally low-tier and do not pave the way for more serious health issues.

## Causes of the Common Cold

The Mayo Clinic reports that the common cold is caused by over one hundred different viruses. The most common perpetrator, however, is the rhinovirus. The rhinovirus is very contagious; causing sniffles and sneezes all throughout much of the world during the winter months. Note that the rhinovirus, along with many of the other some one hundred cold-causing viruses, attacks most readily during months with lower humidity. The lower humidity in the winter months brings a greater affinity for these viruses and for the common cold.

## Symptoms of the Common Cold

If you have the cold, you have the following symptoms:

**1. Sneezing**
**2. Stuffed nose**
**3. Fever**
**4. Body aches or headaches**
**5. Fatigue**

6. Cough
7. Sore throat

## What To Do if You Have the Cold

If you discover you do have a cold, look to the later discussed herbal remedies to heal yourself. Furthermore, note that colds are contagious for the three initial days of your illness. Therefore, it's essential that you stay home and rest to save everyone else from your virus.

## What is the Flu?

Flu, also known by its official name, influenza, is a respiratory illness, much like the cold. However, the flu paves the way for a serious disease called pneumonia. This occurs most readily in older people, in young children, and in pregnant women.

The cold finds its way to people nearly all months of the year; however, the flu is generally seasonal. It runs its course from mid-fall to mid-spring, and it catches the most people during the very height of winter. The flu is captured much the same way as the common cold: through contact with other people with the virus.

## Causes of the Flu

The flu is created, generally, by either influenza A or influenza B virus. These strains can alter, based on the year, leading to the creation of a brand new flu vaccine every single year. Note that the flu vaccine is a very dangerous element—one that should be avoided. We will discuss this in greater depth later.

## Symptoms of The Flu

Flu symptoms include:

1. **Chills and/or a fever**
2. **A hacking, dry cough**
3. **Headache**
4. **Body aches**
5. **Sore throat**

**6. Serious tiredness, lasting up to three weeks**
**7. Runny nose**

Note that many of these symptoms are much like the cold symptoms. However, flu symptoms are much more pronounced and can occasionally result in diarrhea and vomiting.

## Four Most Essential Flu Facts

With the flu season in full swing, it's important to understand the following facts to ready yourself for the months ahead.

### 1. Flu is very contagious.

A person with the flu virus can spread his flu via talking, coughing, or sneezing. What's more: those tiny droplets of "virus" can actually spread about six feet in all directions. Therefore, even if you keep your distance from a flu-ridden person, you might not be far enough away.

Watch out for children, especially. They are the notorious holders and spreaders of the disease.

**2. Flu is one of the more dangerous diseases, and it affects literally everyone: children, older people, and middle-aged people.**

Many people think they're "safe" from the flu. That is: they think because they exercise, they eat correctly, and they stay away from children, they're completely void of problem. However, it's important to remember that more than 200,000 people are affected with the flu virus to the point of hospitalization every single year. Therefore, it's not a disease to be waved to the side. It is very serious.

**3. Another year, a different flu virus strain.**

The flu consists of a viral-based infection with a very unpredictable viral strain. Therefore, every year can bring a brand-new strain of the disease, one that we can't prepare for. Some seasons are far more dangerous than other seasons; unfortunately, these seasons are impossible to predict.

## 4. Flu can seriously hinder your life enjoyment.

This might be a bit of a no-brainer. However, it's essential to remember that when you have the flu, you're completely "out" of your life. Every single year, children miss almost forty million days of school and approximately four million sporting events. Adults report that they miss seeing their family members—especially during this time of year—and that they miss the routine of their former lives. Those seven to ten days of a flu-ridden body attempting to heal itself can really take a chunk from your personal time.

# How to Protect Yourself Naturally

A recent study at the University of Arizona notes that it takes only four hours in a sick-riddled office for common surfaces, like copy machines, to begin brimming with disease. Therefore, you must begin to wrap yourself in protection from colds and flus immediately to ward off fevers, coughs, and continual unrest. You don't want to miss out on anything over the holiday season; imagine watching the New Years' ball drop from your bed at home. Doesn't sound fun, does it?

## 1. Stop drinking alcohol.

If you're a consistent drinker, consider losing the alcohol when you're especially susceptible to colds and flus. Alcohol decreases your ability to fall into REM sleep; when you don't get enough sleep, you are far more likely to catch the cold or the flu.

## 2. Sanitize—everything.

Everything that is touched by many human hands over a period of a few hours—from the microwave to the refrigerator, from the buttons on the elevator to the armrests on chairs, should be sanitized and wiped down every two days during cold and flu season.

## 3. Turn to hand sanitizer—or vodka.

If you don't have hand sanitizer around your house, rub a bit of vodka on your hands to ward off germs. This way, you can completely eliminate germs in the next few hours. (Make sure not to the take a swig, though. See number 1!)

## 4. Don't inhale in the area of a sneezing or coughing person.

This takes a bit of practice. The next time you see someone sneezing or coughing, casually "breathe out" until you can get about ten feet away from him or her. This way, you won't inhale the contaminated air in his vicinity.

## 5. Consider always having your own pen.

How many pens do you casually pick up during any given day? You sign something at the grocery store, at the bank. You have to borrow a pen to make a note at the coffee shop. You pick up a ton of spare germs each time you use a different pen. If you just keep your own—or two—with you every time you leave your house, you could be saving yourself from the cold or flu.

## 6. Rinse your nasal passageway.

Consider rinsing out your nose to get all the "gunk" out of there and help yourself breathe easily. Do this by mixing together 1 teaspoon of baking soda with 4 tsp. of iodide free salt. Take 1 teaspoon of this created mixture and mix it with pre-boiled, coiling water. Flush your nose out with this solution to feel comforted and reduce your interior germs that could ultimately result in a future bodily illness.

## 7. Stop touching so many things.

That's right. How many things do you casually touch during the day? Do you utilize the hand railing on the stairway? Do you turn to drinking fountains for water? Maybe avoid doing these things during the next few months of flu season. Bring your own water bottle until, say, May.

## 8. Go get a massage.

I know, I know. It's probably not too hard to convince you to go treat yourself. However, a massage can boost your bodily circulation, which can release extra nourishment to all of your cells. This reduces your feelings of stress, which in turn boosts your immune system.

## 9. Sweat toxins out.

In a later section, we'll discuss the great benefits of exercise on your body to ward off sickness and disease. However, it's essential to really stick this into your skull: you have to sweat toxins out of your body in order to feel better and ward off disease.

## 10. Get eight hours of sleep.

If you're at great risk of developing disease right now, try to get extra hours of sleep. If you get around eight hours of sleep per night, your body will boost an extra bout of immunity in order to attack all lurking viruses.

## 11. Wash your hands often.

This is a no-brainer, perhaps. However, it's essential to wash your hands continually throughout the day and then always pat them completely dry. If you allow your hands to "air dry" they can become dry and flaked. This provides an open passageway for germs.

## 12. Regularly clean your cell phone.

You're always touching your cell phone, bringing it up to your mouth, and taking it with you everywhere. Keep an extra batch of sanitizing wipes with you everywhere, and always wipe down your phone between uses. This can seriously cut down on your risk of disease.

# Chapter 2
## THE FLU VACCINE:
## THE CONTROVERSIAL TOPIC

Ah, yes: the topic of flu vaccination. This brings a very controversial issue, indeed, with many people on both sides spouting their beliefs about its effectiveness. Let's look at the facts, discuss the issues at hand, and make an informed decision about whether or not the flu vaccine is an essential element on the road to good health this flu season.

Note that during the 2012 winter season, the flu vaccine was found to be effective only fifty-six percent of the time. This percentage point was drawn across all age groups. However, a look at the older, senior age group reveals an even darker point. Only nine percent of flu vaccines received by seniors over the age of sixty-five were shown to be effective.

These numbers force us to reconsider the flu vaccine.

There's a great deal of propaganda involved with the flu vaccine. With the coming flu season, both doctors and the media work to promote flu vaccines; but throughout their advertising mission, they fail to mention all the harm that flu vaccines cause. Note that you cannot rely on your doctor's advice, or the advice of the "popular agenda" of the population to make decisions about your health and your child's health. You must educate yourself about what's available.

Side effects of the flu vaccine include muscle soreness, bodily discomfort, Guillain-Barré syndrome—which consists of nerve damage, increased risk of flu infection, disability, and even death.

While it's pretty uncommon to die from the flu vaccination, it's also very uncommon, actually, to die from the flu.

Generally speaking, flu-related deaths are attributed to bacterial pneumonia; at their core, bacteria are dealt with utilizing antibiotics, respirators, and parenteral antibiotics. Viruses, on the other hand, must run their course, which they can do naturally in a healthy body, void of the flu vaccine.

Furthermore, all vaccines are pulsing with poisonous chemicals that are immediately injected into your body. Some of the chemical-based ingredients currently added to vaccines today are:

1. **Antifreeze**
2. **Formaldehyde**
3. **Sulfates**
4. **Acetone**
5. **MSG**
6. **Yeast proteins**
7. **Glycerin**

There's further evidence that vaccines are grown in both human and animal tissues such as monkey tissue, chick embryos, and human diploid cells.

When you inject these chemically-laden vaccines into your bloodstream, your body doesn't have an ability to process them correctly. This would be different if you actually ate them. During the digestion process, the body has the chance to eliminate toxins from your food. However, once these toxins enter your bloodstream, the damage enters into every cell of your body.

Other parts of the world are currently altering their vaccination laws and experiencing decreased death rates. For example, Japan raised its age of vaccination to two years old, disallowing babies younger than this from receiving vaccination. As a result, their infant mortality rate decreased substantially. Currently, they're #3 on the lowest level of infant mortality rate, while the United States ranks in at #33—an embarrassingly high rate of infant death.

Furthermore, in April 2010, Australians halted their flu vaccinations in children under the age of five. Many, many children landed in the emergency room with convulsions just a few hours after their vaccination, leaving Australia in a brief state of vaccine-related emergency.

## A Better Way to "Vaccinate"

A flu vaccine actually exists in the natural world—without the utilization of a scary, artificial vaccine. In fact, vitamin D—an element found most readily in sunlight— can boost the immune system and force the body to create CD8 T cells, which are, essentially, white blood cells that attack antibodies and pathogens at a cellular level. Therefore, a "cocktail" flu vaccine might not need to be created if the entire world looks to vitamin D for more vibrant immune systems.

But how will vitamin D work against a tried-and-true body criminal, the virus?

Essentially, research shows that just because your body has a virus in its midst, doesn't mean that you will get sick. If your body is continually operating at its optimal efficiency, it can handle a few viruses and pathogens swimming around, without trouble. Vitamin D, itself, can create many antimicrobial peptides that battle against viruses and fungi—thereby assisting your already revving immune system.

It's further essential to note that about sixty percent of all the children who died from swine flu—H1N1 in the 2009 epidemic, had other health problems, such as cerebral palsy, epilepsy, or other neurological disorders. All of these immune and neurological disorders are further linked with vitamin D deficiency. This was probably linked to the children's high susceptibility to the H1N1 disease.

## How to Get More Vitamin D

It's essential to get enough vitamin D in order to create your own natural flu vaccine. Look to the following ways to achieve this endlessly beneficial vitamin.

1. Get yourself in the sun.

Sun forces your body to create vitamin D. Try not to overdo it, of course, as the sun can damage your skin cells and create mutations. Aim for around twenty minutes of non-sunscreen exposure per day.

Note that if you're older, have a darker tone to your skin, or if you live in higher latitudes, you will need to seek other routes to achieve the correct amount of vitamin D.

2. Increase your intake of omega-3 fatty acid fish.

To increase your vitamin D intake, consider eating an extra dose of tuna, salmon, trout, or eel. (Omega-3's are really good for your heart and brain, as well!)

3. Increase your intake of mushrooms.

When mushrooms are exposed to light, they experience the same reaction as humans: they create vitamin D!

Despite the fact that many mushrooms are grown in the darkness, you can look to Portobello mushrooms for an awesome

400 IUs of vitamin D in each 1-cup serving.

## Damage from a Vaccine Can Never Be Undone

If you delay your flu vaccination decision, you might be doing yourself a favor. You're allowing your immune system to do the work for you; thus, you're allowing your immune system to strengthen itself without the necessary help from the vaccine. Furthermore, you're allowing your child's immune system to bolster up a bit, which is a really essential process during his or her developmental years.

When you have a vaccine, however, you cannot undo it. Therefore, if you can do without it and still avoid the flu—why wouldn't you?

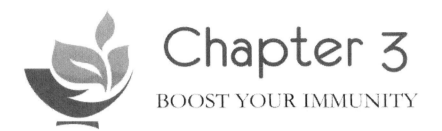

# Chapter 3

## BOOST YOUR IMMUNITY

## What Is Your Immune System?

Essentially, your immune system is the element of your body that notices and fights back against viruses, bacteria, and other foreign substances in your body. You were born with an innate immunity. This formulates an initial line of defense, which includes your skin, stomach acid, your ability to cough when you inhale a foreign substance, the enzymes lurking in your skin oils and your tears, and your the mucus in your nose.

If a pathogen goes beyond this initial defensive line, it is attacked by your acquired immunity.

Acquired immunity is an evolution of your immunity that has grown around its exposure to entering antibodies. Therefore, it has learned how to beat foreign pathogens, and it will again.

The blood components of immunity include specific formations of white blood cells, blood proteins, and chemicals. "Lymphocytes" is the correct term for white blood cells. A typical immune response is made up of B and T lymphocytes. B lymphocytes produce attack-ready antibodies that attach to pathogens in your body and thus "target" them for later destruction. T lymphocytes, on the other hand, attack those already targeted pathogens and further release cytokines, or chemicals that bring ultimate control of your immune response. Note that when you prick your finger, for example, T lymphocytes send out cytokines that bring the immune response to that prick; as a result, your finger is inflamed. Your body is attempting to heal itself. It's showing an immune response in action.

Once T and B lymphocytes are formulated in your body to attack, they generally multiply to create memory T cells and memory B cells. This allows you, for example, never to get the chickenpox again. Your body remembers how to respond.

How is your immune response? Recent research states that your affinity for colds, flus, and other illnesses during this sickness season depends on how strong your immunity is. If you find yourself continually with a sore throat and a runny nose, you might not have an ability to heal yourself and fight back against pathogens on a cellular level.

**Learn about five additional signs of your inability to have an appropriate immune response:**

**1. You eat too many sugary sweets.**

When you eat too much sugar, your body has a difficult time metabolizing it. Essentially, you put on weight—which on its own can have various side effects such as an increased risk of diabetes. However in addition, research shows that if you eat about one hundred grams of sugar, your white blood cells are unable to kill any pathogens during the five or six hours after this sugar-inhalation. Therefore, if you eat a bunch of candy canes and then retreat into the world of flu and illness, your body will not be able to fight against the germs you picked up on the stair railing or on the drinking fountain.

## 2. You don't turn to water and other liquids.

When you're sick, you require fluids. This is something you probably hear from your doctor all the time, right? Note that if your pee color is not a pale yellow, you aren't getting enough fluids to flush toxins out of your body and help your immune system reboot. Reevaluate your water intake. Aim for 8 glasses of filtered water per day.

## 3. You weigh a little bit extra.

If you are overweight or obese—with a body mass index of over 40—you have an impaired immune system. This extra weight forces your body into a hormonal imbalance. This fuels inflammation that halts your body's immune response.

**4. You have high stress levels.**

How often do you catch a cold directly after your most intense and stressful workweek? Note that chronic stress, or long-term stress, automatically forces your body into a lowered state of immunity.

**5. You turn to well water for your hydration needs.**

You're trying to get extra bouts of fluids. That's wonderful! However, if you turn to well water for this hydration, you might get sick. Research shows that more than twenty-five million people from the United States drink well water; furthermore, this well water contains more arsenic than is considered "safe to drink." Note that the arsenic further distracts your immunity from dealing with the cold and flu viruses, thereby putting you at greater risk of picking up the diseases.

## Herbal Remedies to Strengthen and Boost Your Immunity

Work to renew and create a more vibrant, healthier immune system with the following herbal remedies. As you work through the following herbal remedies, it's important to remember to get enough rest, to eat healthy, unprocessed foods, to maintain proper hygiene, and to reduce your stress levels.

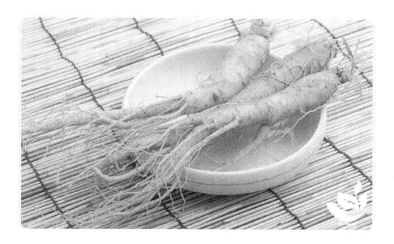

### 1. Ginseng

Ginseng is a Korean-based herb with an active ingredient called ginsenoside, which fuels both anti-cancerous and anti-inflammatory properties. Research shows that this herb can boost your immune system and further lower your stress levels.

Note that ginseng cannot be found in any food-based sources.

Alternately, find ginseng tea at your local health food store.

# Ginseng Tea Recipe

### *Ingredients:*
3-inch piece of ginseng root
Water
Honey

### *Directions:*
Begin by peeling and slicing the ginseng root. Next, pour honey to coat the ginseng root and allow it to sit out for twenty minutes.

During this time, heat the water to near-boiling temperatures. Pour the water over the ginseng in a mug or a bowl and allow the root to steep for ten minutes. Afterwards, strain the water and enjoy the tea.

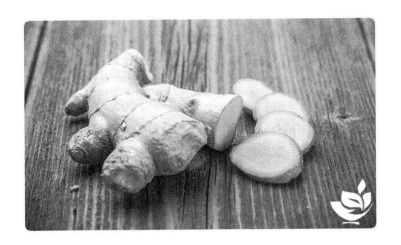

## 2. Ginger

Ginger works to reduce your body's overall inflammation, your risk for blood clots, and your level of cholesterol. With this reduced state of inflammation, your white blood cells have the ability to focus on other things in your body—like pathogens, for example—rather than continually focusing on your body's chronic inflammation (formulated by the foods you eat and the lifestyle you create).

Ginger can be found in tea or capsule formation.

# Ginger Tea Recipe

### Ingredients:
Two-inch piece of ginger root
3 ½ cups water

### Directions:
Begin by peeling and slicing up the ginger root.

Next, allow the water to boil in a saucepan. After it begins to boil, toss the ginger root into the mixture and allow the water to simmer for twenty minutes.

Afterwards, strain the tea and brighten it a bit, if you like, with lemon.

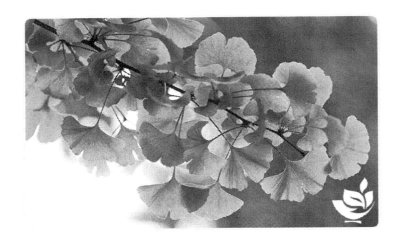

### 3. Gingko Biloba

Gingko biloba has leaves with incredible antioxidant elements called ginkgolides and bilobalides. These elements protect your body from free radicals, which work to create inflammation that ultimately leads to cell death. When your body is no longer hindered by a continued state of inflammation, your white blood cells can focus more readily on the flu season at hand.

Note that gingko biloba can be found in capsule or tea formation.

# Gingko Tea Recipe

## Ingredients:
1 cup water

1 tsp. gingko leaf

## Directions:
Begin by bringing the leaves into a small bowl. Next, pour the boiling hot water over the gingko leaves. Allow the leaves to steep for eight minutes. Next, strain the water, and drink the tea. Add a bit of honey or lemon to sweeten the rough flavor.

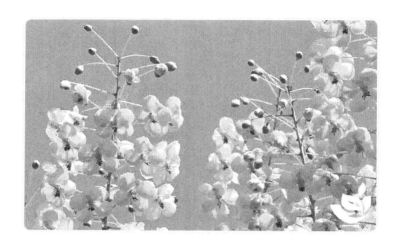

## 4. Cat's Claw

This Peru-based herb is often utilized for stomach disruptions. However, recent research has shown that it boosts the immune response on an undeniable level. It wards off degenerative diseases and common infections, like the cold. Furthermore, it boasts a number of oxindole alkaloids, which actually allow your immune system to have a better ability to "swallow" and destroy pathogens.

Note that cat's claw can be found as a supplement or as a tea at your local health food store.

# Cat's Claw Tea Recipe

*Ingredients:*
Bark or ground cat's claw
Lemon juice
Water

*Directions:*
Begin by boiling a cup of water. Pour the boiling water into a mug, and drip a bit of lemon juice into the water. The lemon acid releases the essential tannins.

Next, add 2 tsp. of ground cat's claw in a tea strainer to the water. Alternately, position two medium-sized bark pieces in the tea strainer.

Allow the cat's claw to steep for ten minutes. After ten minutes, drink the tea, adding a small bit of honey, if you like.

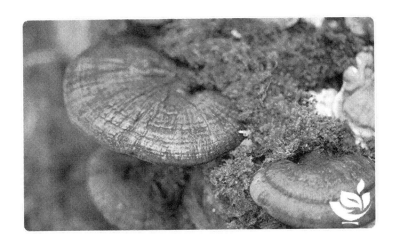

## 5. Ganoderma

China-based ganoderma is a popular medicinal herb that fuels greater health and longevity. It both fights back against cancer-causing free radicals and boosts your immunity. Furthermore, it is pulsing with antioxidant elements.

# Ganoderma Tea Recipe

## Ingredients:
5 grams dried ganoderma, also known as reishi mushrooms
water

## Directions:
Break the reishi mushrooms into pieces. Note that they're quite difficult to break apart, and you might need to utilize your hands or a heavy blade.

Bring a pot of water to a boil in a ceramic or a stainless steel pot. Drop the reishi mushrooms into the boiling water and reduce the heat to create a simmer. Allow the mushrooms to simmer for two hours.

Next, strain the water and allow the liquid to cool down. Drink the tea warm. If it tastes too bitter for you, you can add a bit of green tea or a small drop of honey.

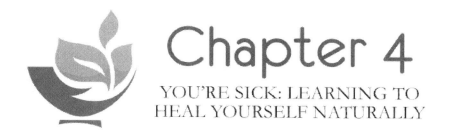

# Chapter 4

## YOU'RE SICK: LEARNING TO HEAL YOURSELF NATURALLY

It happened: your immune system was down. Your body was caught off-guard, and now you're sniffing, sneezing, aching, and feeling miserable.

Look to the following herbal remedies to heal yourself naturally, assist your immune response, and feel better more quickly.

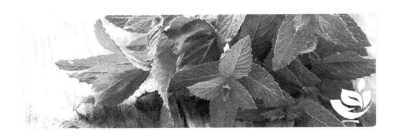

## 1. Relieve Your Aching Head with Peppermint

Peppermint tea can relieve one of the most troublesome elements of your cold and flu: your constant headaches and body aches. Furthermore, this tea works to sooth any stomach discomfort you have.

*Ingredients:*
½ cup chopped peppermint leaves
1 ½ cup boiling water

*Directions:*
Begin by chopping up the peppermint leaves. Place the leaves in a tea bag.

52

Next, boil the water, and pour the hot water over the tea bag. Steep the peppermint leaves for ten minutes. Then, drink the tea with a bit of honey or lemon, and feel the waves of calm pass over you.

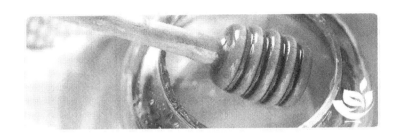

## 2. Sooth Your Cough with Raw Honey

Raw honey is pulsing with antibacterial, antiviral, and antifungal elements. It further soothes your aching throat and relieves your cough.

### *Ingredients:*
2 tbsp. raw honey
1 ½ tbsp. coconut oil
1 tsp. cinnamon

### *Directions:*
Begin by melting the coconut oil either in the microwave or in a double boiler. Then, mix the coconut oil with the cinnamon and the honey to create a paste. Eat the paste throughout the day, every time your throat begins to hurt once more.

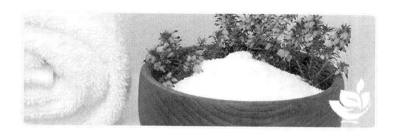

## 3. Boost Your Circulation with an Epsom Salt Bath

Baths can do more than relieve your chronic stress. This Epsom salt bath can boost your circulation, allowing nutrients and white blood cells to circulate more readily in your system and fight your illness.

*Ingredients:*
½ cup Epsom salt

*Directions:*
Pour the Epsom salt into your warm bath and sit as long as you like, inhaling and exhaling the wonderful salty scent.

## 4. Make Your Own Vapor Rub to Breathe Easily

If you're having trouble breathing as a result of your terrible cold or flu, you should look to this DIY vapor rub. This particular recipe is much better than the store-bought variety because the store-bought kind contains processed crude oil and toxic turpentine.

*Ingredients:*
3 tsp. beeswax, grated
8 tbsp. coconut oil
3 tbsp. Shea butter
20 drops lemon essential oil
20 drops rosemary essential oil
15 drops eucalyptus essential oil

*Directions:*
Begin by melting the Shea butter, beeswax, and the coconut oil together in either a double boiler or a glass bowl positioned over a boiling pot of water.

After the two ingredients melt together, remove them from the heat and add the essential oils. Pour the Vaseline into a sanitized mason jar (or another sealable container). Utilize the Vaseline to place on your temples, nose, cheekbones, or your chest to breathe easier during the day and night.

## 5. Natural Remedy Cough Salve

If your cold or flu is assaulting you with a myriad of coughs, look to this natural cough salve remedy to soothe your throat and bring regularity to your breathing.

*Ingredients:*
3 tbsp. beeswax
6 tbsp. coconut oil
1 tbsp. olive oil
20 drops rosemary essential oil
10 drops tea tree oil

*Directions:*
Begin by melting together the coconut oil and the olive oil in a double boiler or in a glass bowl positioned over a boiling pot of water. After the ingredients begin to melt, add the beeswax and stir well.

Next, remove the mixture from the heat and add the essential oils. Allow the mixture to cool a bit, and then pour it into a sealable glass container.

Utilize this cough remedy by rubbing the salve over your feet and then placing socks over the salve. Sleep like this through the night to relieve your night coughing fits.

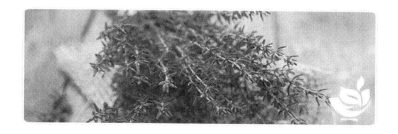

## 6. Throat Soothing Thyme Tea

Soothe your aching throat and bring ready relief with this herb-based recipe. Note that thyme is an herb that actually makes your coughing more productive; therefore, it works to "heal" you through coughing, rather than keep you in constant strain.

### *Ingredients:*
10 ounces boiling water
2 tbsp. fresh thyme leaves
½ tbsp. honey

### *Directions:*
Begin by boiling the water. Place the thyme leaves in a bowl or a mug, and pour the water overtop. Allow the leaves to steep for six minutes. Afterwards, strain the water and add the honey to the hot

tea. Relax and inhale; drink the tea and feel better.

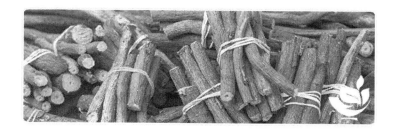

## 7. Licorice Root Tea to Fight the Virus

Licorice root contains an element called glycyrrhizin. This element is a powerful antiviral, even against SARS and HIV. Furthermore, it's been noted that licorice can fight back against flu and cold viruses quite easily.

### *Ingredients:*
8 ounces water
2 tsp. dried licorice root

### *Directions:*
Begin by boiling the water in a saucepan. After it begins to boil, add the licorice root to the water. Remove the pot of water from the stovetop and allow the licorice to steep for ten minutes.

After ten minutes, strain the tea and toss out the root. Drink the tea warm, and enjoy.

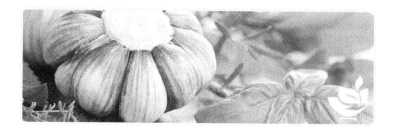

## 8. Chew on a Clove of Garlic

If you want to relieve your cold and flu symptoms, you should chew on one clove of garlic, per day. It not only boosts your immune system and relieves your aching throat but also fights back against the virus currently working its way through your system.

Note that it's not proven whether or not cooked garlic has the same effect. However, if you enjoy the flavor of garlic, adding a bit to your cooking will not hurt you one bit; in fact, it may provide medicinal benefits.

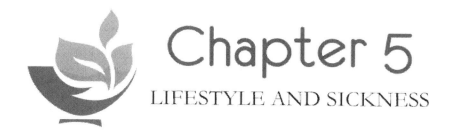

# Chapter 5

## LIFESTYLE AND SICKNESS

The way you live your life can seriously affect your risk for disease and your ability to fight back. Note that as aforementioned, you should always get enough rest, drink plenty of fluids, eat good, unprocessed foods, and try to get a bit of exercise to sweat out the toxins. Read on for more extensive information.

## The Importance of Diet

The connection between what you eat and your risk of illness leads us to that initial, thousand-year-old saying by Hippocrates: "Let thy food be thy medicine and thy medicine be thy food."

Research shows that the profound alteration in the way people ate in the twentieth century created a modernized increase in chronic illness. Therefore, it's essential to eat the following foods—not just to heal yourself from disease, but to further create a healthy, strong body that can ward off future pathogen invasion.

## The Importance of Protein

If you're sick with the cold or the flu, you must eat plenty of good, healthy protein to keep your body in top shape and to build strength. When you eat protein, especially from poultry, lean meats, dairy, legumes, seeds, and nuts, you're further honing in on nutrients like vitamin B6 and B12; both of these nutrients create a more efficient immune system.

Furthermore, protein sources are rich with both zinc and selenium, which create strength for your white blood cells and your immune response.

## The Importance of Flavonoids

Flavonoids are, essentially, phytonutrients that bring vibrant color to fruits and vegetables. Research notes that the highest concentration of flavonoids exists in citrus fruits, such as oranges, grapefruit, limes, and lemons. These flavonoids strengthen your immune system.


## How To Load Up on Vitamin C

Doctors proclaim the importance of vitamin C in the wake of cold and flu season. It's important to remember that vitamin C actually cannot prevent these colds. It can, however, halt your illness in its tracks a good deal ahead of time, allowing you to enter back into your life once more.

Oranges are the poster children of vitamin C intake. But did you know that oranges don't actually have the most vitamin C count in the known vegetable and fruit universe? Check out the following "superfoods for vitamin C health" in order to load up on vitamins, supercharge your immunity, and reduce the duration of your illness.

## 1. Red Chili Peppers

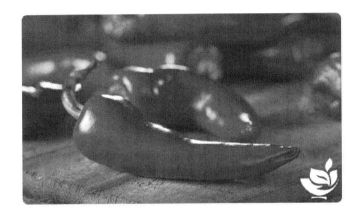

Just one half cup of red chili peppers fuels you with 108 mg of vitamin C. Furthermore, capsaicin in red chili peppers can actually relieve your bodily aches and pains, which are natural symptoms of both cold and flu. In addition, capsaicin helps to thin down respiratory mucous so it's easier to cough up expel mucous secretions.

## 2. Green Peppers

Just one cup of green bell peppers lends you 120 mg of vitamin C, which is double your normal daily recommended vitamin C allowance. Furthermore, green peppers are pulsing with fiber, which can help you become more regular and expel toxins.

## 3. Broccoli

Cancer-fighting broccoli packs 132 mg of vitamin C per cup. Furthermore, it's very low in calories, making it an essential stop on your road to weight loss.

## 4. Papaya

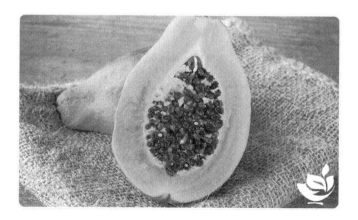

Delicious papaya is revving with 88 mg of vitamin C. Furthermore, it's been shown to clean out your sinuses and make you look bright and youthful on the outside. In other words, you can end your sickness and look even better than you normally do if you eat papaya.

**5. Brussels Sprouts**

Little balls of Brussels sprouts are absolutely delicious when roasted. Look to them if you want 75 mg of vitamin C per one cup serving.

## The Importance of Exercise

Exercise lowers your risk of catching colds and flus. Just thirty minutes per day can seriously boost your immune system and fight back against bacterial and viral infections.

Essentially, when you exercise, white blood cells fly through your body far more quickly, fighting against all the viruses and bacteria as they go along. Furthermore, exercise lowers your stress levels, which decreases the amount of free radicals in your system. When your body has a decreased level of free radicals, your body's inflammation levels lower; as a result, your immune system can pay closer attention to actual, exterior pathogens attempting to enter your body.

Furthermore, when you exercise, you automatically improve your ability to get adequate amounts of sleep at night. As mentioned previously, getting at least eight hours per night is crucial to keep your immune system in fighting shape.

Unfortunately, you should not turn to extreme exercise if you want to ward off sickness. Marathon trainers can substantially weaken their immune system (because they are essentially creating extra inflammation in their body as they run for multiple hours). Furthermore, extreme weight lifting can deplete your white blood cells and increase your stress hormone levels.

When should you exercise, and when should you stay home?

Essentially, you can do light exercise if you have either the cold or the flu and you DO NOT have a fever. A fever is a sign of deeper damage. It's essential that you stay hydrated as you exercise and listen to your body, stopping whenever you need to rest. Note that the flu is very contagious; therefore, if you can avoid exercising at the gym, you could save a lot of people some serious hardship.

## Anti-Sickness Supplements

Look to the following anti-flu, anti-cold supplements to heal yourself, reduce your symptoms, and decrease your illness time.

### 1. Zinc

Zinc is very essential for your immune system to work properly. Furthermore, when you take zinc as a lozenge, it can reduce your cold symptoms such as cough and runny nose.

## 2. Vitamin D

If you're vitamin D deficient, look to a vitamin D supplement, like Source Naturals Vitamin D-3 Drops or Vitacost Baby D's for an extra 400 IU per drop. Remember the importance of vitamin D, as outlined in a previous chapter. Vitamin D could further help decrease your risk of developing the flu or the cold in the future.

## 3. Vitamin C supplement

Vitamin C is very important for your immunity to work properly. While you can consume enough vitamin C through the previously mentioned vitamin C-rich foods, you can further find Vitamin C in supplements like MedlinePlus and Nature Made Vitamin C in your local health store for an additional boost.

## Conclusion

Natural Remedies for Colds and Flu walks you through all the essential elements of getting through your cold and flu season safely. When you understand the symptoms of both the cold and the flu, the differences between them, you will live your life differently to avoid them. Furthermore, this book works to give you the real facts in a very propaganda-laden world about the flu vaccine. Decide for yourself whether or not to get the vaccine, but understand the undeniable toxins currently lurking in the man-made product.

Find yourself healing and boosting your immune system with all of the essential herbal and natural remedies mentioned in this book. Heal your aching throat and your pulsing head; reduce your overall cough and fever symptoms. Promote circulation, and begin to bolster your immune system to halt your illness in its tracks.

You can heal yourself and live more naturally this cold and flu season. Don't allow this truly annoying and very life-debilitating disease ruin your day-to-day life.

21431386R00045

Printed in Great Britain
by Amazon